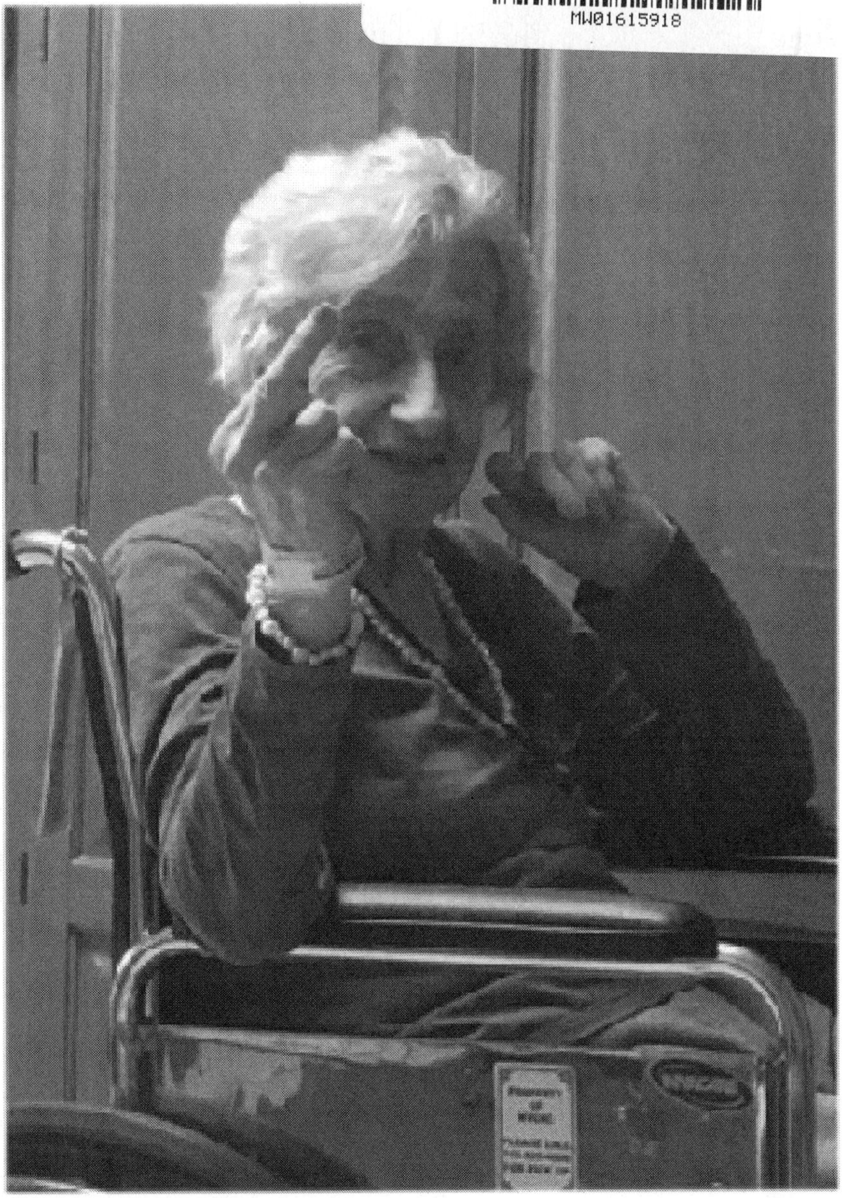

#ShitMyMamaSays

A humorous look at life while dealing with dementia.
In loving memory of my Mom, Mary Lou.

My Mom

Mom

I guess there's a lot to be said in this part because Mom is the catalyst for me writing my first cookbook/memoir, *Escape To Ravioli Mountain - A Memoir in Food*. Even though a lot of the focus in that book is primarily about my time living with my grandmother in the 1970s, it doesn't take away from the fact that Mom was always an inspiration. No kid comes with an instruction manual and no parent goes into parenting knowing everything. Once you understand that, it helps you really grasp what kind of parenting you grew up with and how you survived through the years where your parents really didn't know what they were doing but did their best. That being said, there's the adage that the parents that you see in their old age are not the people you grew up with. You're looking at old people who are trying to get into Heaven. That also being said, I feel like my mother and I have come full circle—from my small beginnings in Pennsylvania, to her needing me at the end of her life in New York. We have always remained very close friends and spoke every single day until the end.

In 2015 Mom moved in with me and my partner. After many years of living with my brother in Florida, she had become our new roommate. By that time, Mom had signs of advanced dementia: She was forgetful, repeated herself a lot but was as sweet as ever and she never argued with me. We were best buddies who cooked together, watched TV, and—when I went to work in the evening—my partner would take over Mom duty when he got home from work. They became besties too. My partner had just lost his mother to cancer when my Mom moved in. It wasn't healing for him, he hadn't really even had a chance to mourn his own mother and suddenly became a part-time caregiver again. My cousin Lynn and I often joked that we "shared custody" of Mom at this time. It wasn't until Lynn called me telling me that Mom set fire to the microwave while trying to cook baby carrots that I knew there wasn't much time until she'd need to go to a nursing home. Imagine my cousin's face when her kitchen was full of smoke with smoldering baby carrots in the microwave. I wasn't prepared for the task of helping an elderly parent adjust to life in the city. Eventually, things got more serious and Mom became seriously ill quite a few times—and fell a lot at home. After a pulmonary embolism almost took her from us, we opted for her to remain in a nursing home as a permanent resident. This was probably the hardest decision I have ever had to make. The anger, the fear, the uncertainty of my mother's voice while she was adjusting to her new home was gut wrenching. I wouldn't wish that pain on my worst enemy. As a child, you never want to disappoint your parents. I thought, in some way, I had let her down. When she was moving up here she was a little scared but I picked her up at the airport and that was some small comfort. I remember we sat in my cousin Lynn's house and I poured us two fireball shots and we toasted and said we were gonna get through this together! And with that, we both did shots for the rest of the evening until my cousin Lynn came home and found us passed out on the couch. I'll never forget that day because it was a day that I took my personal needs and put them all aside to figure out how to take care of the situation and do what would be best for Mom. That was probably one of the most grown-up things I've ever done at that point. However, I didn't do it alone. Mom spent time with my cousin Lynn, and my cousins Debbie and Carol. She also spent a lot of time with my nieces Karen and Kathy in Florida. I wasn't prepared for Mom living with me, and there aren't enough thank yous I can send to my cousins who helped me by taking care of Mom during that period. She was passed around from relative to relative until, one day, I had no choice; she had to move in with me and I had to take responsibility for her. My Mom had survived so much and then—in her later years—was forced to let the bank foreclose on her house—the property that she had grown up in and the house and property that I had growing up in! Dementia took all that away, and eventually she'd end up in a nursing home. The nursing home that I chose for Mom was based on my location. Not exactly the worst location and not exactly the best, but it was 12 blocks from my home and it was easy to keep tabs on her. The staff members there were lovely, sweet, generous and kind to her. I visited often and, pretty soon, everyone got to know me. Her favorite nurse was named Paul. He was very sweet and was her best buddy at the home. He was also the person that I confided in and could basically get the truth of the situation from. He talked fast because he didn't like to stay on the phone, but when I saw him in person we had many chats about my mother's care. Being in a nursing facility is not for the faint of heart. In the time that Mom was there, six people died and they were all friends of hers. I watched her deteriorate along with them. The worst was when her best friend Josephine passed away. Even though Mom was dealing with the throes of dementia and she was aware enough to call me and say "Josephine quit. She's not going to work here anymore." So I took that as her way of dealing with the loss and in her mind Josephine was off to another "job." It was better than her dying. My last images of Josephine were painful. This was a very sweet woman who was in a wheelchair, who had very bad sores on her legs from diabetes and other ailments. She was crying and she reached out to me and said "please take me home! Are you here to take me home?" And Mom echoed the same sentiment. "Yeah, take us both home. She can stay upstairs and I can stay downstairs. We'll get an elevator put in the house." Meanwhile, the house she was referring to had been foreclosed on over nine years before, but we took this and put on a brave face. You need to smile to always make them feel like their reality is real and not question it. When you put on a brave face, you smile until the elevator door closes. That's usually when I would start to cry—from the elevator to the hallway to exiting the building to either walking home or getting a cab. Most of my visits to Mom would end in smiles at the elevator and tears on the way home.

The joy that Mom brought to me and many people— THAT was priceless. Her #ShitMyMamaSays posts are her own epic words, and I posted them on social media. It was my way to cope with the situation, to share and connect with others who may have had similar situations and could maybe identify with this as it may have been how they coped as well.

In February 2020 Mom started to have weird symptoms. Everything from gastric issues to breathing and coughing and nausea. She went to and from the ER a few times between January and March.

Mom died on March 21st, and I got sick with COVID on March 22nd. It was a blur, honestly. It was incredibly hard. The last time I got to see her was March 10th. She was just getting back from the hospital and I stopped by on my way to work. I'm glad I did. The next day, the governor announced that all visitations would be stopped for nursing homes. We followed up on FaceTime with the activities director. She set up calls daily at 11 am and I got to speak to Mom up to the day before she passed away. Navigating through COVID after a death and getting sick myself was indeed difficult. Sirens 24/7 from March to May. Ambulances driving past my house almost hourly. Makeshift morgues on the sidewalk next to hospitals because they were overrun with dead people. Every funeral home and hospital had refrigerator trucks parked outside and all were filled to capacity because funeral homes and crematoriums couldn't keep up with the demands. I was supposed to get Mom's ashes back within a week, but due to my illness and the backup at the funeral home, it was six weeks before she was finally cremated and I was well enough to get her ashes. I haven't looked at the urn since it arrived, and the ashes are still in a cabinet and will be buried next to my dad in the summer of 2021—on her birthday. I wish I had the words to thank everyone who helped me with Mom over the past six years—including those who were instrumental in helping me work through my grief. You get one mother in this life and I cherish every moment I had with her. We said "I love you" at the end of every visit and every call. I still remember her hugs and her voice. I also saved many of her messages on my voicemail. Her message was simple:

> *When you have stress, anger or frustration, laugh.*
> *Find a way to laugh and find a way to make*
> *everyone else laugh. I hope that you enjoy the path*

we went on as mother and son and I hope that you get a chuckle out of our story.

Maybe you have a relative with dementia, or someone in your family recently became a resident at a nursing home. This can be a very difficult time. It's my hope that this book will help you—guide you and give you a chuckle, because everyone needs a little #ShitMyMamaSays! Try reading one quote per day or read the whole book in one sitting. The ultimate purpose of this book is to give you a daily laugh, but choose your own path!

--With much love, Bobby Hedglin-Taylor

March 21, 2021

Handing Mom a glass of water at the nursing home…

"I don't drink Water. Fish fuck in it."

Mom: Bobby can you turn down the air conditioner? I'm freezing my guyoonz off!

Bobby: What the hell is a guyoon?

Mom: I don't fucking know, but they're cold.

In the elevator at Mom's nursing home, she points to a gentleman standing beside us…

"He's my lover."

Mom: Bob, we're going to see a Broadway show tomorrow!

Bobby: Wow that's great Mom. What show?

Mom: Something, something Mexican with Chita Rivera. It's called Miss Saigon.

Just back from seeing Kinky Boots—a musical with drag queens—on Broadway, Mom asks…

"The show was fantastic but, Bob, those were guys, right? So, where do they put their things?"

Not able to let it go, Mom calls me for the fourth time – asking me to explain how drag queens "tuck."

"Bobby, they use duct tape? Won't that rip their pecker off? It's definitely got to rip off some hair!"

Mom: Happy Birthday Bob!

Bobby: Thanks Mom. It was yesterday.

Mom: Really? Are you sure?

Bobby: Yes Mom. I visited, and we called my cousins and watched TV, and shared some chocolate peanut butter cakes.

Mom: Oh yeah that's right and your cake gave me the shits!

Mom: Bobby, who gave me all this chocolate?

Bobby: Susie and Deb.

Mom: Do they know it gives me the shits?

Bobby: Well, they've read this, so now they do!

Looking at a picture of a friend's new baby…

Mom: Who's the father?

Bobby: She was artificially inseminated. She and her wife chose the donor.

Mom: So the father's not involved?

Bobby: No.

Mom: Oh that's much better when the father's not involved. What a beautiful baby.

Mom answering my cousin Lynn who asked if she was watching *How to get away with Murder?*

"No. That would give me too many ideas."

Calling Mom from the line to get into Burning Man—an annual social/self-expression experiment in the desert. She got excited and shouted to her friends at the nursing home...

Mom: Bobby just made it to the desert with 70,000 boy scouts!

Bobby: Not quite Boy Scouts, Mom, but let's go with that.

Calling Mom on April 16, 2017…

"Happy Thanksgiving, Bobby!"

Checking up on Mom…

"Bob, I'll have to call you back. I'm playing…
[yelling into the phone]
BINGO!!!!!!!!"

…Mom won $2!

Mom: Bobby, I need some Tums.

Bobby: Mom, I just bought you a whole bottle two weeks ago.

Mom: I ate them! What the hell did you think I did with them, put them on my salad as fucking croutons!?

Sometimes Mom hoards soda. She hands me three six-packs of ginger ale...

"Bob, take this soda. I can't drink it. I'll piss my brains out!"

Bobby: Mom, why do you have 20 boxes of tissues?

Mom: Shhh! Hide them!! I'm building a stash!

Asking if she needs anything before I come visit…

"Don't forget to bring me some Depends.
I'm all out and the diapers here squash my bug!"

"Bobby, I love chocolate, but do they make chocolate that doesn't give you the shits?"

Mom: Bring me a pair of scissors.

Bobby: Why?

Mom: The hair on my bug is too long. I need to cut it. It's so long I can braid it.

Bobby: You've asked for a watch, hairspray, and now a pair of scissors. When the nurse asks me about it, what am I going to tell her? You're sprucing up your vagina?

Bobby: Mom, where is your phone?

Mom: [grabbing her boobs] Right here between the only two suckers I can trust.

Mom: We had a singer today, Bob.

Bobby: How was he?

Mom: He couldn't sing for shit.

Bobby: Was he that bad, Mom?

Mom: A fucking cat in heat would sound better!

Mom got into trouble at the nursing home.

Bobby: Mom, what happened?

Mom: She turned me in to the big boss and said I called her "a fucking bitch." I've never used that word in this fucking place before, but Bobby, she IS a fucking bitch! Anyway, I've never used that goddamn word here. I need you to get on your computer and fix my resume so I can get a new job and get the fuck out of here.

Handing mom a chocolate peanut butter cake...

"No thanks. I'll just shit my brains out."

Bobby: Mom, would you like a coffee?

Mom: Are you fucking crazy? I'll be pissing my brains out.

"Bob, I just had a fight.

The bitch hit me first!"

Hoarding A&D ointment…

"It's great for your heinie."

"How do you tell that the president is lying?

His lips are moving."

Looking at a photo of a very pregnant friend.

"Oh she could go anytime!
Tell her to just dangle a BBQ chicken wing down there to coax him out.
It worked for you, Bob."

Mom: Why did I change my clothes?

Bobby: Mom, you were wearing this when I got here.

Mom: You're crazy, I was in a white pantsuit and now I'm in jeans!

In her mind, my Mom is Hillary Clinton.

While singing along to "God Bless America" at the home, Mom sings…

"God bless America, and fuck you Trump!

I get off the elevator at the home and the room next to Mom's is buzzing with activity—nurses are rushing in and out of Mom's room. She looks up at me and says…

"Bobby, what the fuck did you do?!"

A patient is moaning in the cafeteria.

Mom: I'm gonna choke the living shit out of her!

Nurse: MaryLou, it is not very ladylike to choke the living shit out of someone.

Mom: You wanna bet?!

Mom was getting her nails done when I was visiting...

Mom: Bob, I gotta pee!

Bobby: Mom, be careful you'll smudge your nail polish.

Mom: Oh, shit. I'll get pink nail polish on my flower.

Mom left a voicemail at 2:30 AM…

"Bob, you gotta get me out of here. I want to go back to Pennsylvania. The nurses here are all a bunch of assholes. Oh, and bring me a box of depends."

Bobby: Hello lady!

Mom: Why the fuck are you always so happy?

Bobby: Buongiorno Principessa!

Mom: Who the hell are you calling princess?

Bobby: Mom, you keep rushing our visit. Do you have a date?

Mom: Yes, I have a date with a fig on Prune Street.

"I love watermelon but if I eat any more I'll be pissing my brains out."

Hiding cutlery in her wheelchair seat…

"You never know when you're gonna need this shit."

Telling Mom I am working on Broadway Bares—a benefit with sexy dancers—to raise money for people with HIV and AIDS…

"Oh, you were always good with animals."

At Christmas day dinner, Mom addresses a fellow patient...

"You are a castrating bitch.

Merry Christmas."

Bobby: What are you up to?

Mom: What do you want? I'm busy. They got me making fucking necklaces!

Bobby: What color?

Mom: Green, and it won't go with any fucking thing I have!

Bobby: Oh, I gave you a nice green blouse for Christmas.

Mom: Oh, that's nice. I better go before the boss comes back."

Mom: I got a big fucking pimple on my bug!

Bobby: Let the nurse help you.

Mom: But Bob, I got a huge pimple ON MY BUG! It hurts like hell! If it was on your dick you'd understand!

She's not wrong.

Mom sitting with her favorite nurse, Paul.

Mom: Hi Bob. OH SHIT!!
I gotta Piss!
[she slams the phone down on the desk and I hear the nurses yelling.]

Nurse: Mary, I'm going to help you!

Mom: Fuck you! I'm pissing myself!

Later the same day…

Bobby: Hi Mom, how are you doing today?

Mom: Great Bob. HOLY SHIT! I'm gonna piss myself again!

She slams the phone down.

Sitting with Mom but on the phone with work…

Bobby [on phone]: We need a pickle to control the chain.

Mom: Why the fuck do you need a pickle in the circus?

Bobby to Mom: A pickle, in rigging terms, is a motor remote control to fly people.

Mom: What is it? Like a dick?

I was touched she finally remembered I worked in the circus industry.

Mom: I have to take my pills earlier, they don't make me tired.

Bobby: The nurses give them the same time every day.

Four minutes later...

Bobby: Mom, are you awake? [She snores] OK, I'm going. Goodnight. [I turn off the TV.]

Mom: Bobby, why are you turning off the TV? I was watching that!

Bobby: Mom, how are you doing?

Mom: I'm in the elevator.

Bobby: Why are you in the elevator?

Mom: I met a guy and we are fooling around in the elevator.

"These male nurses are nice but, when they help you in the John, I warn them:
What you're about to see is **not** new."

Mom: Bobby, check my sneaker. There's something in there.

Bobby: Mom, it's a Corn chip!

Mom: WHEN THE FUCK DID I EAT CORN CHIPS?

Mom: Bobby you work too much!

Bobby: That's life mama!

Mom: Tell your boss I think you work too much and they don't want me to come down there.

Bobby: OK Mom, right away.

Bobby: Another cup of coffee?

Mom: I'll piss my brains out!

Bobby: Like what our bodies should do when we drink?

Mom: Do you want a cane in your head, smart ass?

Bobby: Two sugars and milk?

Mom: Sure…I like that new almond milk.

As the phone rings…

Mom: Bobby, what's that noise?

Bobby: Your boobs are ringing again.
[Grabs her chest, gets the phone out of her bra and looks at the phone.]

Mom: Oh fuck, it's your cousin. Tell her I'm at work.

Seeing a commercial for a sex lubricant on
LOGO, Mom asks me…

"How do you use BOY BUTTER?"

Mom to me: Hey Red!
I'm sweating my ass off.

Walking out of church one day, Mom was just not having it…

"Immaculate Conception? Bullshit! Mary got fucked! If you kids want to stay here and listen to this bullshit, be my guest."

Mom noticed some extra pills with her breakfast…

"What the fuck is this? Did you rob a pharmacy!?"

Raising the shades in her room, the reflective light from disco-ball Christmas ornaments on her tree bounces across the room…

"Don't bring them up too high, just bring the blinds up until your balls are resting on the ledge."

"Mario Cantone is gay?

He's a nut.

I never knew he was gay. I thought he was normal!"

"Why am I taking Prozac? I'm with my son. I'm happy! I don't need that anymore."

Passing rather loud, uncontrollable gas while visiting my mother…

Mom: What did you say?

Mom: Bobby, what's this?

Bobby: It's ice water, Mom.

Mom: Ice water?
Who do I have to fuck to get a
cup of coffee?

A little old man walks by in a robe and walker…

"Now that one—he's just looking in here to see if I'm naked!"

Mom: What did the doctor say I had?

Bobby: It's called pancreatitis.

Mom: Well, I call it '*hurts-like-hell-and-shitting-my-brains-out*!'

Mom: Did you bring my hair brush?

Me: Yes Mom.

Mom: Good. Now give it to me! I look like a 50-cent whore who was out all night!

Mom on nursing home life...

"Jesus fucking Christ! Ninety percent of the people in here are old!"

Watching *Swamp People* on TV…

"Hot damn! I wish I was there huntin' gater!"

#LookOutAnnieOakley

Me cleaning mom's drawer…

Bobby: You have about 30 packets of A&D ointment here.

Mom: Bobby, take that home.

Bobby: Sure, Mom. I use it on my tattoos.

Mom: I use it on my rectum.

Hearing about where she puts A&D Ointment…

Bobby: TMI, Mom. TMI

Mom: Oh, you want to change the channel to watch the TMI channel? It's channel 68.

Bobby: You mean TLC Mom?

After seeing *Jersey Boys*, the musical…

Mom: Those guys must have had a lot of face work done! They look really young and those guys are my age!

Bobby: Mom, That wasn't the real Frankie Valli and the Four Seasons. They were actors.

Mom: Still, they were great! Especially that little Frankie.

Seeing mom was not feeling well after eating too much Halloween candy, I lifted the cushion from her wheelchair and found it was full of peanut butter cups…

Bobby: Why do you have all this candy here!?

Mom: I'm building a stash.

Asking her about the pain she was experiencing…

"The pain is down there. You know —where my bug is."

Mom: When's your birthday?

Bobby: It's tomorrow.

Mom: Ah, Fongool!

Me: You remembered it.

Mom: I can't find my checkbook. I wanted to give you a check.

Me: You don't have to.

Mom: Are you shitting me? I want to make sure you get a present or I'll end up in a home!

Getting caught trying to rip her IV out, the nurse called me and put Mom on the phone…

"What? I wasn't pulling on my IV. That was somebody else! That fucking nurse is full of shit!"

Patient: Nurse, I'm gonna die here!

Mom: People die here every day. Where the fuck have you been?

In the days leading up to her passing, I talked to Mom via FaceTime. Due to the pandemic, the governor shut down nursing home visitations. She laughed a lot, she wasn't sad, she was smiling and that's how I want to remember her, and you should too. Death is not the end. Even though she's not physically here anymore, you now have her words, her jokes, and all the #ShitMyMamaSays to help you through your own path. Life is funny and you should always find a way to laugh no matter what. Life goes on and Mary Lou is in my heart and memories forever. I loved sharing her with you.

Thank you for taking this journey with us.

DEDICATION

This book is dedicated to my mom, all the families of the people who were lost in the pandemic and to all of the front line health workers.

Thank you:
- Mom for being my mother, my best friend and for your amazing humor and spirit.
- The staff at The New York Center for Rehabilitation and Nursing, especially Paul and Marilyn. She loved you both very much.
- The incredible Debra Chilcott
- My editor, EJ SEPP
- Lynn Shea, Joe Mackin, Debra Weidman, Susan Campbell, Charles Weidman, Carol Coco, Jack Weidman, Elizabeth Streb, Christine Chen, Sarah Boyce, Rebecca Fey, and my brother Howard Hedglin for their love and support.
- A huge thank you to Suzie Sims Fletcher for her incredible friendship, mentorship, editing, guidance, love and support during this process. None of this could have been possible without Suzie!
- David Andrew Taylor, whose love and support made this possible.
- Thank you Barb Drozdowich. Your guidance and knowledge is so appreciated!
- Finally, to everyone who encouraged me to write, compile and share mom's quotes. That love and support really made this possible.

Because she would like you to laugh, I saved this one for last: Mom on death…

"Bob, when you're dead you're dead. If you can't afford to bury me, just stick a beef bone up my ass and let the coyotes drag me away."

In loving memory of
Mary Lou Hedglin
August 7, 1937 - March 21, 2020

When it rains, it's not sad, it's the angels crying with joy because my Mom and #ShitMyMamaSays is making them laugh.

Laugh.

Every day.

Even if your heart is breaking.

Peace out, until we meet again.

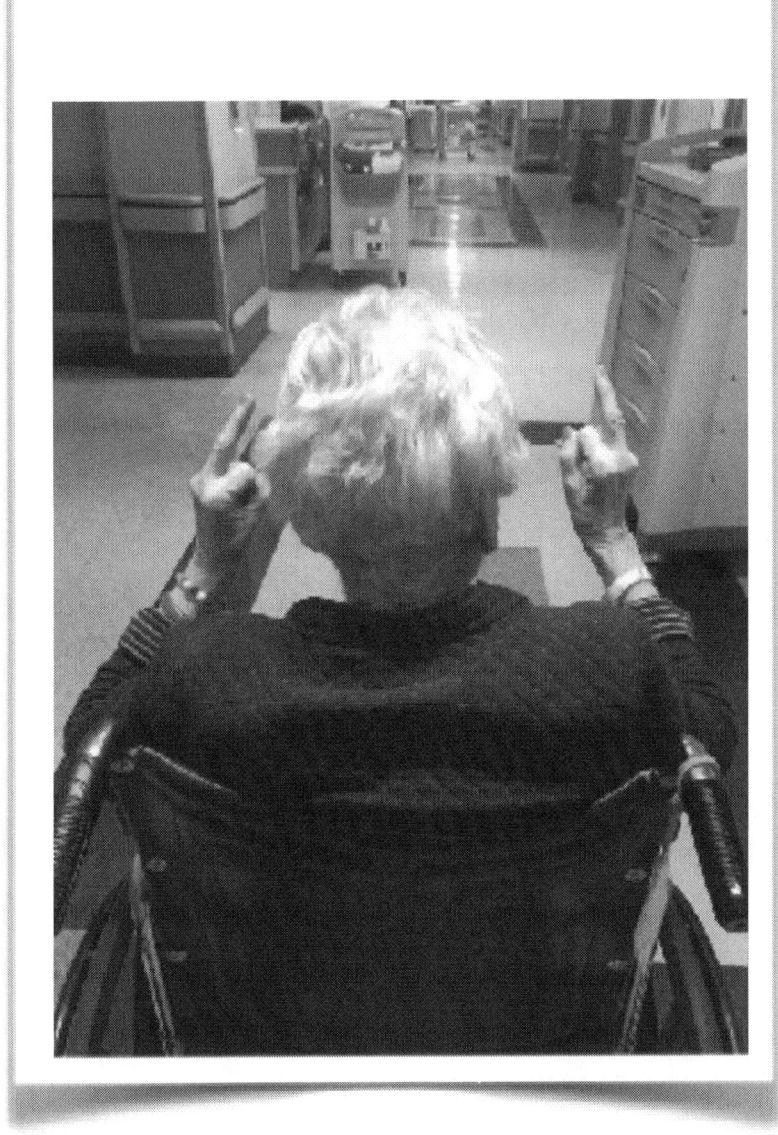

99001711R00055